If hypertension can be diagnosed and treated by the methods outlined in these pages at an early stage, rapid recovery can occur without any complications. The same methods, if followed assiduously by long-term sufferers, will produce a slow drop in blood-pressure, while disastrous end-effects such as cerebral haemorrhage and arterial sclerosis can be largely avoided.

GW00686379

Nature Cure for High Blood-Pressure

J. Russell Sneddon N.D., M.B.N.O.A.

THORSONS PUBLISHERS LIMITED
Wellingborough, Northamptonshire

First published 1955
Seventh Impression 1971
Second Edition, revised and reset, 1973
Seventh Impression 1983

ISBN 0 7225 0224 9

Printed and bound in Great Britain by
Richard Clay (The Chaucer Press) Ltd.,
Bungay, Suffolk.

Contents

I.
Nature Cure and High Blood-Pressure

HIGH BLOOD-PRESSURE CAN be termed one of the modern ailments, and it is usual to find that the condition is associated, at least in the lay mind, with mental and physical strain. It is easily appreciated how this thought arises, for during the past twenty years most people have undergone considerable nervous strain, and the term, which covers the group of symptoms called high blood-pressure, is now commonplace, whereas previously it was very rare. Undoubtedly, nervous strain has, in many cases, something to do with the raising of blood-pressure, but it is not the whole answer.

This ailment is usually associated with middle and old age, but it also occurs in youth. When it does arise in the teens, it is probable that there has been some systemic poisoning such as bowel toxaemia, pyorrhea or excessive smoking. At middle age, the general finding is that businessmen and housewives are frequently affected. It is easy to understand how the harassed businessman can build up a certain amount of tension, especially neck tension, which upsets his digestive powers and increases the nervous contraction of his arteries. In the case of the housewife, many cases of this ailment arose during the last war, when the housewife was inclined to deny herself the proper foods to enable her family to be adequately fed. Allied to this were the worries of running a home efficiently under wartime conditions.

It is not generally known that this trouble, or at least the tendency to it, can be inherited, but statistics have proved that it seems to run in certain families. This often means that there is some specific weakness in the make-up of these people, and usually the ductless glands are affected. It may also mean, however, that children of parents suffering from high blood-pressure are reared in a way very similar to that in which the parents were brought up, and so are subject to the same ill-effects of dietetic errors and wrongful habits of living. Another point of interest is that these children, although they may not have acquired the physical weakness of the parents, may be forced into a state of nervous tension. This can arise from a desire on the part of the parents for the children to become accomplished at something which they them-selves disliked or which they were conscious of an inability to achieve. This forcing of the child who may already have a weakness or a predilection towards high blood-pressure can cause the onset of the trouble. This point must be studied carefully by all parents.

High blood-pressure can arise as a primary condition, that is, it does not need to be associated with disease in any other organ. In these cases some disturbance of the endocrine glands, usually the adrenal or pituitary, is suspected, but this is a very difficult condition to diagnose. These are very peculiar findings, but they prove that other organs of the body may be in perfect health as far as the reactions to all test can show, and yet high blood-pressure may be present.

To complicate matters further, it is possible for a person to be seemingly perfectly healthy and yet register a high blood-pressure. This may not be a sign of actual disease, and a considerable study of the person is required before a finding of normal high blood-pressure is confirmed. These people may go through life at a high rate and yet never exhibit any of the signs of strain that appear in the person who is suffering from a pathological blood-pressure. Every case of this nature becomes a special study to the physician. Usually, however, after careful recordings have been made of the condition of the heart, pulse and breathing rate, and of the methods of living of the patient, the diagnosis is made of residual or natural high blood-pressure. In such cases, it is usually found impossible to reduce the pressure to any great degree. The arteries seem to be specially strengthened in these cases to deal with the strain, and the heart also has a great power of compensation for the excessive effort required from it.

Usually, however, rising of the blood-pressure above the normal is a sign that other organs of the body have been overworked and are becoming distressed, the customary belief being that ill-health only shows in the second line of defence of the body. The initial organs may be disturbed for years without showing definite signs, and it is only when the second line of defence of the body becomes disorganized that symptoms of ill-health make their appearance.

WARNING SYMPTOMS

These symptoms, in high blood-pressure, are often very fleeting: an occasional headache, giddiness, a desire to be always working and forcing the body onwards. Intermixed with these come moments of extreme tiredness in which, without seeming exertion, the patient feels physically incapable of effort. Digestive upsets are also common. It is usually believed that the person who suffers from high blood-pressure has a tendency to a florid complexion, but although this may be an associated symptom at the beginning of the trouble, as the dangerous stage of blood-pressure is reached it is customary to find that the patient becomes pale and rather drawn-looking. When this change occurs it is likely that the pressure has reached a serious stage.

Many sufferers from high blood-pressure are not aware that the pressure is exceedingly high, and the first real sign is when the arteries collapse under the strain. The person then suffers from extreme weakness, and when the blood-pressure is taken it is found to be very low. Low blood-pressure is a common end-result of high blood-pressure, and the condition is always a serious one. It is preferable, in every circumstance, to begin the treatment of high blood-pressure before the entire system collapses, because when this occurs the treatment is necessarily very much prolonged.

In Nature Cure, the patient himself is responsible for regaining and maintaining health. Certainly, the path can be made clear and guidance can be given on the various steps by a Nature Cure practitioner, but the actual healing force within our bodies is the one essential to good health. No one can give this healing force, although the practitioner may be able to make it more vital and enable it to flow more freely. Every treatment must fail if the healing force within the body is not brought into action, and the whole theme of this book is the strengthening and releasing of the healing vitality of the body. By so doing, the greatest of all factors in the restoration of health is being employed. Without it, health on any level is impossible; and yet it is the common finding of most Nature Cure practitioners that people are so unaware of the healing force which lies within the body that they do everything, or seemingly everything, to destroy it or to reduce its potentiality.

VITAL HEALING POWER

Throughout the following chapters, this basic idea must be kept in mind. We are trying, in everything we do, in our change of diet, exercises, care of the skin, and in our mental and emotional outlook, to release the vital healing power. Nature alone heals, and she heals through this inherent power that is present in greater or lesser degree in every one of us. The people who suffer from high blood-pressure are usually those who have a certain amount of nervous and physical vitality; indeed, in many cases it is said that they have too much vitality. This means, of course, that these people, if they follow the Nature Cure system, become well fairly quickly, because the healing force is at a high level. In most cases, Natural Healing means a reduction in the amount of expendable vitality; in other words, these people are slowed down by this method and so are enabled to live much longer and in a considerably greater degree of health than would normally have been their lot.

This slowing down of their activities comes naturally with the reduction in the energizing foods on which these people live mainly. This must not be regarded as a sign that the treatment is not being successful, because the reverse is true. Whenever sufferers from high blood-pressure undertake treatment which reduces the pressure, they tend to become tired and listless. The explanation is that the body is carrying out much of its own cleansing and, while it is doing so, it does not want to expend energy on physical needs.

The treatment, if followed assiduously, will result in a slow drop in the blood-pressure, but it is impossible in every case to promise that the normal pressure for the patient will be obtained. Most people take up Nature Cure when all other methods have failed, and in some chronic cases a full recovery may be very difficult to achieve. In nearly every case, however, a reduction of blood-pressure becomes slowly apparent, and disastrous end-effects, such as cerebral haemorrhage or severe arterial sclerosis, are very largely avoided. On the other hand, if the patient becomes aware early that he or she is suffering from hypertension, the methods outlined in this book will bring about a rapid recovery without any complications whatsoever. The treatment described in this book is natural and basically sound, and it can be undertaken with the utmost confidence by anyone suffering from high blood-pressure.

2.

The Arterial System

OUR BODIES CONTAIN a great network of arteries and veins which radiate through all tissues, supplying food and removing the end-products of combustion. In the study of blood-pressure it is the arterial part of the blood system that is the most important, and the path of cure is easier to understand if the reader has some idea of its working.

The main arteries begin at the heart, where they are very large. They then decrease in size, until at the distal parts of the body, such as the head and feet, they are approximately only one cell thick. The arteries are in continual movement and have a much stronger construction than the veins; an extra muscular coat allows them to contract and expand in relation to the beats of the heart. When the heart beats strongly the blood is pumped in a surge through the artery, which enlarges slightly as a result of the pressure. The heart then relaxes and the artery contracts because of its elastic nature.

This means that the flow of blood is kept more or less continuous by this interaction between the heart and the arterial wall. The arteries never close completely because of the amount of blood contained in the system, and a certain pressure of blood is always present. It follows, therefore, that everyone has a blood-pressure, although it must be understood that, in practice, this pressure is only recorded in the larger arteries. When the more distant parts of the body from the heart are reached by the arterial flow, the blood is oozing rather than flowing into the tissues.

SYSTOLIC PRESSURE

Two important blood-pressures are studied by Nature Cure practitioners investigating a case of arterial tension. The first is that recorded in the large arteries when the left ventricle — that is, the large pumping chamber of the heart — has contracted and with its powerful action forced the blood into the arteries. This naturally causes an increase in the blood-pressure already in the artery and this, the highest pressure recorded, is called the *systolic* pressure.

This is the reading usually taken as important in all cases of high blood-pressure, and in medical circles it is reckoned that it should be roughly one hundred plus the age of the person; that is, a person who is forty years of age should have a pressure of one hundred and forty. In the practice of Nature Cure it appears that this guide is too high; recordings of blood-pressure on a balanced system of living will be given later.

The systolic pressure varies from the normal in accordance with changes in the structure of the body, but when it is very high it always betokens one thing, namely, that the heart is being strained excessively. A high pressure also means that the heart, although being strained, is strong. This is naturally a good thing; and when the strain on the heart is relaxed, recovery can be rapid.

The heart is a specialized form of muscle, and is extremely strong because of the work it has to do during its lifetime. Its action is so arranged that the period of rest is equal to or even greater than the period of work, and in normal circumstances this prevents the heart from becoming tired. If it is forced, however, to work against an enormous pressure, the energy expended by the heart is greater than normal and weakness results. The body, recognizing this, compensates in several ways, but naturally the greatest help to the heart is when the blood-pressure is lowered.

A high systolic pressure can also mean that fluidity of

the bloodstream is suspect. There are several causes of this, and the workings of the kidneys, skin and lungs must be examined. In Nature Cure we are concerned with the whole body and not with individual upsets, and each organ must be included in the treatment. When this is done, it can be confidently expected that the bloodstream will regain its correct viscosity.

If, for any reason, the arterial walls have become hardened, the resistance to the passage of blood will naturally be very much increased, and a higher pressure required to force the blood to the distant part of the body. Arterio-sclerosis due to any cause tends to raise the blood-pressure, because the heart naturally does everything in its power to force the blood to every tissue.

So the factors concerned in a high systolic pressure — commonly called high blood-pressure — are the efficiency of the heart as a pumping mechanism, the fluidity of the bloodstream and the state of elasticity in the arterial walls.

DIFFERENTIAL PRESSURE

The second important pressure in the arterial system, at least from the Nature Cure angle, is called the *differential* pressure.

The heart rests between each beat, and in doing so, it harbours its energy so that it can work efficiently for many years. During this resting stage the blood-pressure naturally falls, and the pressure then recorded on the instrument is called the *diastolic* or resident arterial pressure. The difference between the systolic and the diastolic, the high and the low, is called the *differential* pressure. This is very important, because it gives the experienced practitioner a definite clue to the state of the patient's arteries. The differential pressure then becomes as important as the systolic, and in certain cases may even be of more value.

It is generally understood that in adult life the differential pressure should vary between forty and fifty points, and this is a usual finding during the consultation with a person in ill-health. A comparatively new form of treatment such as Nature Cure naturally leads its practitioners to keeping accurate notes of blood-pressure changes, and many interesting findings have been recorded. It has been found that, after a person has followed out for several months the tenets we teach, there is a considerable drop in the differential blood-pressure until it reaches a level of between twenty and thirty points. According to medical standards this pressure is too low and denotes a tiredness or lack of vitality. This is not our finding, and most of our patients are amazed at the vitality and staying power gained during the treatment.

A low differential pressure means a less vigorous circulatory flow, and also decreased tension in the arteries with a reduction in the wear and tear of the circulatory system. In many cases, therefore, the aim of the naturopath is primarily to reduce the differential pressure, by either lowering the systolic pressure or increasing the diastolic. In addition to considerable success in all blood-pressure cases, this treatment is of the greatest value in arterio-sclerotic changes involving arterial spasms which are often diagnosed as actual thrombosis.

If the desired reduction in the differential pressure takes place after the diet and the other factors explained in this book have been thoroughly established, it means that the treatment is proving beneficial in many respects and is not limited to blood-pressure reduction. The heart is not working so energetically and will naturally last much longer, the life of the arteries is prolonged and the danger of circulatory failure is removed.

Here are some examples of blood-pressure changes taken from our case-book.

Mrs C., suffering from stomach ulveration. Age 53.
Blood-pressure at initial consultation:

Systolic .168
Diastolic .94
Differential 74

Although in this case the actual highest blood-pressure was not dangerous, the differential of seventy-four showed severe fatigue of the arteries. After six months' Nature Cure treatment her pressures were:

Systolic. .154
Diastolic .100
Differential 54

This would be termed a normal blood-pressure, but I would have preferred it to have dropped another ten points.

Miss A., suffering from high blood-pressure. Age 45. Blood-pressure at initial consultation:

Systolic .180
Diastolic .138
Differential 42

In this case the high systolic pressure was the trouble, and the treatment advised was very strict. Within three months the pressures dropped to:

Systolic .130
Diastolic .85
Differential 45

It is interesting to examine the blood-pressure of a man aged sixty-eight who has been on a strict Nature Cure diet for twenty years. When he first started this way of life he followed a dietary very much like the one outlined in this book. Throughout the years he found, however, that his body functioned very well on a plain diet, and he became more and more inclined to reduce the quantity of food. At present he has one main meal each day, and for the rest of his diet he takes fruit and fruit juice only. He is a vegetarian and does not drink tea or coffee, and his occupation is a strenuous one involving great physical effort. During the last ten years he has not had one day off work through illness.

His pressures are:

Systolic 128
Diastolic 90
Differential 38

By ordinary standards of reckoning blood-pressure his systolic and differential pressures would be reckoned too low for a man of his age. With this in mind, I lately made a thorough examination of all his reactions and found him in perfect health. His retinal arteries showed absolutely no sign of arterio-sclerosis, and his heart reacted easily to all tests without change of rhythm and the whole system was without strain. Recently he passed a driving test at the first attempt, which shows the efficiency of his nervous system.

Many people become worried when their blood-pressure (systolic) drops below normal and they fear the arteries are collapsing. This condition is only dangerous when the body has become very tired following great physical and mental strain, and a complete rest is then required to bring about a cure.

3.
The Causes of High
Blood-Pressure

IF AN ATTEMPT is made to cure any physical disability it becomes much more simple if the cause or causes of the trouble are fully understood. In this chapter I wish to discuss, without going deeply into medical terms, the various causes of an increase in blood-pressure.

There is a form of high blood-pressure which unfortunately is not associated with any other physical upset, and this is called *essential hypertension*. It arises seemingly within the glandular system, although it may have other associations with certain organs; in spite of all tests it is impossible to determine what is actually upsetting the system. This presents a baffling problem which has been treated from many different angles without any striking result.

In Nature Cure, however, we have an advantage, because it is appreciated that it is impossible to understand everything that occurs within the systems of the body. We also know that if the proper conditions can be created, the healing vitality that is within the body will always attempt the cure. This is a very comforting thought, and it means that we can treat essential high blood-pressure – that is, high blood-pressure without any definite cause – successfully by general Nature Cure methods.

These, although they are applied to high blood-pressure can be used with benefit in every form of ill-health, and they give the Nature Cure practitioner a very great advantage over any other type of practitioner. It is the practitioner's duty to explain how obedience to the laws of nature leads gradually to health through the workings of the healing vitality, and this explanation is the theme of this book. Please notice that this is a lasting but not a quick cure. Very few people understand that they become ill over a period of years; they believe that such-and-such a trouble only started a week or a month before. Ill-health is a progressive state and begins whenever we start ill-treating our bodies. It may be years, however, before serious symptoms become apparent. In these circumstances it is impossible to regain health quickly, but each month of treatment sheds a certain depth of illness, and gradually the patient returns to health. This is what happens in every case of high blood-pressure which is at all curable. A slow but definite improvement is desirable because spectacular cures are seldom beneficial in the long run.

SCARRING OF ARTERIAL WALL

One definite cause of high blood-pressure is some form of scarring of the arterial wall. This scarring is usually brought about by some poisonous matter getting into the blood-stream and causing inflammation. It may be due to poisoning from lead, tainted food or even excessive medication. It can also arise from chronic alcoholism and over-indulgence in tobacco. Whatever the cause of the inflammation, the end-results are always the same, namely, the inner surface of the artery becomes inflamed and when this heals a scar tissue formation is left.

Scar tissue is inelastic and has not the power to expand or contract to any great extent, and if it is present within the arterial wall it is always detrimental. Our arteries depend very much on the efficiency of their elasticity; with each pumping action of the left ventricle of the heart the blood-pressure sweeps through the arteries and causes them to enlarge. The left ventricle then relaxes and the arteries contract, and it is the vitality of this elasticity that makes the artery fulfil this function. That vitality is lost when scarring takes place in the inner wall of the artery.

The artery affected by scar tissue will expand when the heart pumps, but it is a sluggish action and more effort is required by the heart. In the same way the artery affected by scarring contracts when the left ventricle relaxes, but usually it either over-contracts or does not contract enough. There is seldom a happy medium in scarred tissue, and detrimental results always follow when this tissue formation is present. In many cases the whole arterial system becomes scarred, and this is followed by an immediate rise in the blood-pressure. Such cases are usually incurable.

ARTERIAL RUPTURE

Another important point is where the scarring takes place. Usually it is found that where the finer arteries are affected, arterial rupture is common. This is always a weak point in the arterial system, that is, the distal parts of the body, and if any part is going to collapse it will be in this area, unless, of course, there has been tremendous strain on one of the larger arteries. This is one of the reasons why cerebral haemorrhage is so common as an end-result of high blood-pressure. The very small arteries in the brain area become hardened and cannot stand the strain, with the result that blood leaks through the arterial wall in a way that should not be possible, gradually impinging on the brain substance and causing nervous reactions due to pressure.

Impurity or toxaemia within the bloodstream does not always attack the walls of the arteries but affects the nervous system of these vessels. This is rather difficult to understand, but it means that in certain cases the nervous system is more sensitive than it should be and is easily upset by blood changes.

There are, of course, many forms of toxaemia — that is, poisons arising from impurities within our systems — and these were specially numerous after the last war, as a result of the poor quality of food. The result was that most of us took unnatural substances into our bodies, and these poisons upset the nerve endings. This often means, in cases of high blood-pressure, that the nerves controlling the muscles of the arteries become irritated. Our arteries have three muscular coats, and the nerves controlling the circular coat often become over-stimulated and the artery contracts. This contraction may be intermittent or it may always be present, but when it occurs, then the blood-pressure rises beyond the normal.

It is usually found in practice that a nervous contraction due to over-stimulation of these muscles is not so difficult to remove as other causes of high blood-pressure. The irritation may be due to defective teeth, septic appendix, dirty bowel, ineffective kidneys, excessive consumption of tea or coffee or excessive smoking. If the cause of this contraction can be determined, then its removal, combined with a balanced diet, will usually bring about a very satisfactory result. On the other hand, if no cause can be discovered and yet there is definite poor circulation combined with high blood-pressure, this must be termed essential high blood-pressure, which has been discussed previously.

As was stated at the beginning of this chapter, the cause of this trouble lies within the glandular system and is very difficult to determine, but general Nature Cure treatment will allow the body to create its own conditions of cure and bring about a removal of these symptoms. There are, of course, certain emotional causes that bring about a general nervous contraction and a slowing down of the actions of the body, but it is seldom that this general nervousness is so concentrated that it reduces the capacity of the artery. It is much more likely that the arterial nervous system is in direct contact with some impurity that is causing the trouble, and it is along these lines that the cure should be sought.

The last of the main causes of high blood-pressure is over-working of the kidneys. In health, the kidneys act as strainers of the blood and remove water, uric acid, urea and various other salts. When they are working correctly the blood is not allowed to become too concentrated or thickened in any way, but when they are affected the blood is not cleared as it should be and there are, of course, various detrimental substances retained in this fluid.

A sluggish bloodstream means that the circulation is impaired, and with a slow flow, irritation of the walls of the arteries becomes common. Many of the impurities that thicken the bloodstream are actual irritants to the inner lining of the artery, and this in turn sets up some form of inflammation. Here we have a vicious circle, because when inflammation is present the arteries of the kidneys are commonly affected and their efficiency is further reduced.

EXCESSIVE TEA-DRINKING

Kidney weakness is a very common cause of high blood-pressure, and it is mainly caused by over-indulgence in tea, coffee, alcohol and condiments. These substances, if taken in excess, set up an irritation inside the very fine structure of the kidneys and ultimately disturb the blood-pressure. Of all the substances detrimental to kidney action, excessive tea-drinking is the most dangerous, although it is fairly closely followed by the extravagant use of coffee. Tea subjected to prolonged brewing is especially harmful, but when it is quickly infused and receives a small addition of milk it is not so dangerous, because the tannin is precipitated. Anyone who suffers from any type of kidney ailment, particularly if there is some disturbance of the blood-pressure, should stop drinking tea.

The ill-effects of tea are largely accumulative, and it is possible, if the trouble is diagnosed before the pressure has risen very high, to clear the choked kidneys fairly rapidly.

Taking certain fluids and the careful use of the cold compress will do much to bring about a healthy kidney action. The kidneys are very finely constructed, complicated and sensitive organs and have such a cleansing capacity that one organ is able to clean the bloodstream if the other requires to be rested. There is reason to believe that the body utilizes this capacity on certain occasions, that is, it rests one kidney and uses the other for cleansing purposes. This is only an example of the innate intelligence of the body's cells, but it is a guide to us in our quest for health. If we can rest the overworked kidneys instead of forcing them, the body itself will carry on repairing any damage. Certain fluids, however, as already remarked, have a temporary effect on the kidneys, and if used carefully are beneficial; but in the main the cure of kidney trouble, when it is curable, lies in the complete stoppage of the substances causing the irritation and in resting these organs as much as possible.

4.
Fasting and Fluids

THROUGHOUT THIS BOOK each step in the sensible reduction of high blood-pressure will be explained as simply as possible. When the systolic pressure is dangerously high its rapid reduction is imperative, and the methods of achieving this will be detailed in this chapter.

The major dangers of high blood-pressure are a sudden failure of the heart or paralysis due to pressure of blood on the brain. Everyone knows that both these conditions are very difficult to correct, and that even if they respond to treatment, the latter must necessarily be of long duration. So it is only sensible for a person who suffers from high blood-pressure to take immediate steps to reduce it.

When the pressure is extremely high only a very slight disturbance is needed to bring about a serious breakdown, and exertion such as lifting a heavy weight, running for a bus, or even any extreme emotion such as anger, can raise the pressure by ten points and then breakage may occur. This means, of course, that the person who is aware that his blood-pressure is very high should take every precaution until the practitioner assures him that it is not at a dangerous level. Nature Cure is, however, a *whole* treatment; that is, we are not concerned merely with the drop in the systolic blood-pressure but in a general all-round lessening of the strain on the arterial system.

However, the advice given in this chapter is intended primarily to bring about a drop in the systolic pressure, i.e. in the highest pressure recorded when the pump of the heart is fully contracted. Rest is the great thing in this initial treatment, and anyone who suffers from an extremely high blood-pressure is advised to make arrangements for a complete rest of the body. This means, whenever possible, rest in bed, the time being spent mainly in sleeping. People who suffer from high blood-pressure are usually very active, both mentally and physically, and after the first day or two rest becomes very irksome. However, this ruling must be accepted, and a complete rest without even reading is the best of all treatments.

In this connection I like to impress upon my patients that the blood-pressure can be likened to a tall glass tube at the bottom of which is the heart acting as a pump; every time the heart contracts the liquid in the tube is forced up say three feet, and every time it relaxes, the pressure falls. In this way the patient gets a good idea of the terrific strain that is placed on the heart when a very high pressure is reached. Once the patient appreciates that with every day of rest the pressure in the tube comes lower and lower, then he will find this part of the treatment more bearable.

This form of imagination actually does much to create a certain quietness in the patient suffering from high blood-pressure, because it is easily understood. Of course, blood-pressure within the body is not such a simple matter because the elasticity of the arteries and various other factors play a part. Once, however, the patient realizes that rest, in almost every circumstance, will bring down the blood-pressure, then it is much more easily achieved. In addition to rest — that is, actual physical rest — it is also very advantageous if other organs, such as the digestive system and the kidneys, are given less work to do at this time. Naturally, the best way to rest the bowel is to refrain from eating, and this is not so difficult when the person is confined to bed. Fasting of this nature allows the whole of the digestive tract to regain strength and cleanse itself.

EFFECTS OF FASTING

The peculiar effects of fasting must be thoroughly under-

stood, otherwise the patient undergoing this treatment
may become disturbed. Whenever a person who is unused
to fasting begins such treatment, there is, of course, an
increase in hunger, and this must be fought against. This
desire may last for one or two days at a certain intensity,
but afterwards it gradually diminishes. Then various
symptoms arise, not of starvation, as is commonly sup-
posed, but as signs that the body is utilizing this resting
phase to discard impurities. Usually the tongue of an
unhealthy person during a fast becomes very dirty and
discoloured and often very much thickened. It is frequently worse after the first day's fast, and this is a
definite sign that the fast is required. Actually people
should fast, in theory anyway, until the tongue becomes
perfectly clean. In most cases we do not need to go as far
as that and in this treatment we prefer to have frequent
short fasts of a day or two rather than one prolonged fast.
In the latter various conflicting symptoms arise, and in
many cases the signs of starvation appear without the
patient really being aware of them. It requires the
supervision of a trained practitioner to determine when
such fasts should be broken.

So any prolonged fasting should be left to supervision,
preferably in a Nature Cure establishment where the
fasting can be controlled, but in a short fast it must be
understood that there will be definite disturbances and the
tongue will show the above signs. Headaches, and disturbed sleep with dreams and nightmares are common at
this time. All these things mean than an internal cleansing
is taking place in the digestive system, and the body is
throwing out, into the inner side of the bowel, the debris
that has been poisoning the system. These are all very
valuable aids to health. They may be slightly unpleasant
but they are most helpful to the person who is undergoing
treatment for high blood-pressure. When the tongue
becomes very much discoloured it is often advisable to
wash out the lower bowel, using a plain warm-water

enema. This will remove a lot of impurity that has passed down through the bowel and which is being retained to an abnormal degree.

At the beginning of the treatment, however, I think that a one-day or two-day fast is quite sufficient to enable the person suffering from high blood-pressure to bring about some reduction in the pressure, and it is quite common for the pressure to fall from ten to twenty points during this time. Fasting is usually accompanied by the taking of a certain amount of fluid; in many cases fruit juices, because of their cleansing qualities, are advised in quite large amounts. The fruit juice is not an actual food but it supplies minerals, vitamins and cleansing properties that can be utilized in the bowel and also by the kidneys. The sufferer from high blood-pressure, however, usually has overworked kidneys, and it has been my own particular finding that it is better in these circumstances to rest the kidneys rather than force their cleansing.

CURTAILING FLUIDS

Resting the kidneys means that the fluids that are dealt with by these organs must be curtailed. Now during the fasting day or days it is desirable to give some form of liquid because there is, naturally, an inclination for the system to become rather clogged, owing to all the cleansing which is taking place, and water is easily the best liquid. It is a solvent that dilutes many of the more concentrated impurities and at the same time does not invigorate the kidneys to any great extent. It allows these organs to work more slowly than do the diuretics, and yet it prevents the urine from becoming too concentrated.

How much water should be taken is important and, generally speaking, during a fast the thirst should be the guide. Later in this treatment very little liquid will be advised, because too much is liable to increase the volume of blood. Water may 'thin' the blood but it tends to increase its volume, and this is not desirable in high blood-pressure. When resting and fasting, the real guide to the amount of liquid should be the actual compelling thirst that arises, and perhaps several pints of water may be required in the day. On the other hand the thirst may only dictate that perhaps half a pint of water is sufficient. Everyone varies according to the cleansing of the digestive system, and no rule can be laid down except that the thirst should be allayed.

Fasting during a period of complete rest of one or two days will do a great deal to reduce the blood-pressure, and the drop will be accelerated by taking no other fluid than water. Certainly other methods can be practised at the same time, but during this course of home treatment we propose to concentrate on the most simple factors which are, of course, most easily overlooked, and these two methods will immediately affect the blood-pressure and bring it down so many points.

TIREDNESS SIGN OF SUCCESS

When a person suffers from high blood-pressure there is a great tendency for the body to be driven. There is a restlessness, a desire for movement and achievement, and the body is worked on and on. The person feels vital, and during the treatment this period of rest is not usually very much to his taste. As the blood-pressure falls, as it will within these two days, the person will also experience a certain depression of spirits. After the fast the body seemingly becomes tired. This is not really the case; what has happened is that the pressure that has been driving the body on, and using up nervous energy when it should have been resting, has been reduced, and the tiredness is a sign that the treatment is achieving its object. Generally, the pressure will continue to fall until a stage is reached in which the body has rested sufficiently to regain strength, when the pressure will be much lower and the patient will be out of danger. It is a most important stage in the treatment, and this depression of spirits and seeming loss of physical energy must be expected; otherwise, of course, if the patient has no warning of it, he will naturally assume that this is not the treatment for him. Once this stage has been achieved, then the definitely dangerous stage of high blood-pressure has been passed and the stage of healing and rejuvenation of the arterial and heart systems has begun.

Two years ago I was consulted by a man who was suffering from very high blood-pressure. He was fifty-two years of age and had been in charge of some very important work during the war and now was in a responsible post in the engineering world. He was inclined to worry considerably about his work, and he took very little leisure. Six months before visiting me, he had trouble with his kidneys and suffered greatly from swelling of the thighs and ankles, and at the same time his blood-pressure had been examined and a pressure of systolic 252, diastolic 170, differential 82, had been discovered. This was a very serious condition, and he was given certain drugs and rested in bed for three months, during which time the pressure dropped to systolic 212, diastolic 150, giving a differential of 62. This was the lowest pressure that could be obtained by medical methods, and when he went back to his doctor after working for a month he was advised to retire as the kidneys and arteries were in such a poor state that his blood-pressure could never be reduced. When he visited me he was in a very serious state. His blood-pressure had again risen to about systolic 248, diastolic 170, differential 78. This showed that in spite of all the treatment and rest, his condition had improved very little.

It was decided to undergo a course of Nature Cure treatment, and the patient was put to bed and fasted, the duration of the fast being suggested as three days. The first day he suffered, mainly in the afternoon, from a very severe frontal headache, which is usually associated with the bowel, and had rather a restless night. In the morning it was found that his tongue was very much coated, his breath foetid and the frontal headache persisted. During the first and second days he took about two pints of water, but these were the only liquids given, and on the second day he was given a three and a half pint warm-water enema which brought away a considerable amount of bowel debris. By the third day his tongue had cleared slightly, and although there was a great deal of flatulence he definitely felt better, although there was a marked form of depression in which he was inclined to become very negative about his prospects of recovery.

The blood-pressure was then taken and it was found to be systolic 218, diastolic 152 and differential 66. This was a helpful sign, and, although he systolic and differential pressures were still very high, it implied that there was a good chance of a fair recovery. These facts were stressed to the patient and the reason for the depression of spirits explained, and he became determined, as the Nature Cure treatment seemed so logical, to carry it out to a conclusion.

5.
The General Diet

FOR MANY YEARS Nature Cure practitioners have taught the value of balanced dieting in the maintenance of good health. Lately some support in this endeavour has come from the medical profession, but much remains to be done; and because of the intense use of chemicals in the soil and in food we must exercise considerable care in the choice of food.

Experience of many cases has proved conclusively that food has a very important part to play in the health state. Some people will point to the exceptions of this statement, but if investigation of any case is continued it will be found that the offspring of such a person are seldom healthy. Careful dieting, on the other hand, can result in an increase in health throughout the various generations of a family. We are not meant to live in ill-health, and if foods are well chosen the standard of health definitely rises.

There are two main classifications of food for practical purposes. In the first large group come the proteins, starches and fats, and these can be termed the building and energizing foods. They are largely acid-forming, and are usually taken in too liberal quantities. The proteins are eggs, cheese, peas, beans, lentils, flesh foods, fish and milk. The starchy foods are all the grains, starchy vegetables such as potatoes, and fruit such as dates. The fatty foods are butter, margarine, nut oils and olive oil. The subdivisions of this classification should be studied carefully, because their understanding makes arranging a suitable diet for high blood-pressure a simple business.

Into the second large classification of food come the fruits and vegetables. Actually these have very little food value, but they are employed to supply the body with mineral salts, vitamins and also some roughage, all of which are essential to the real health state. Their presence allows the other digestive actions to take place normally. There are many practitioners of Nature Cure who believe that it is not possible to obtain health by dividing food into these two main classifications, and they think that only one-third of the diet should consist of proteins, starches and fats, the remainder being made up from vegetables and fruit. This may be perfectly correct in many cases, but the difficulty of administering this type of feeding makes it unhelpful to most of us.

BENEFICIAL FOODS

The most beneficial foods in all cases of high blood-pressure are vegetables, taken either raw or conservatively cooked, that is steamed or baked in such a way that the mineral salts and vitamins are preserved as much as possible. Fruit in every form is helpful in high blood-pressure, but if there is any accompanying acidic condition such as rheumatism, stomach acidity or the like, it is a wise plan to omit the very acid fruits such as lemons, grapefruit, sour oranges, rhubarb and plums, even if they are tinned. Vegetables and suitable fruits are safe foods in high blood-pressure, but a small proportion of protein is necessarily required for good health; this can usually be taken, without adverse effects, in the form of peas, beans, lentils and in small amounts of egg or cheese. The starchy foods are also essential but must be taken in small quantities. The best forms of starch are baked or steamed potatoes, wholewheat bread and crispbread. Sugars should be chosen from honey, Demerara sugar, treacle, and the sugar-starches such as raisins and dates.

The danger foods in high blood-pressure are all white-flour products; that is, everything baked with white flour, including, of course, all patent flours and manufactured puddings. White sugar and all sweets made from manufactured sugar should also be avoided. Condiments and preserves, especially vinegar, excessive salt, all fried and greasy foods and meat extracts should also be stopped. Meat of all kinds and fish are not advised in this treatment.

The safe liquids in high blood-pressure are water, buttermilk or yogurt, fruit juices provided they are not too acid, vegetable soup, cereal and yeast beverages. I have said that these liquids are safe, but actually it is not advisable to take much liquid in this trouble because the volume of blood must be reduced. The diet should, therefore, be as dry as possible.

There are, of course, times when it is necessary to give some form of liquid; for instance, people on a very dry diet find that the urine occasionally becomes very concentrated, and then liquid is required. Usually in such cases yogurt or some form of buttermilk is of benefit at this time. But even then the amount of liquid taken into the body should be curtailed below the normal to enable the kidneys to be rested and to allow some of the excessive fluid to be drawn from the bloodstream.

HARMFUL LIQUIDS
Certain liquids are definitely harmful in cases of high blood-pressure. All wines, beers, and spirits come within this category; if these are taken freely, the reduction of high blood-pressure becomes practically impossible. Owing to their effect on the digestive and nervous systems the use of such liquids can often bring about arterial blockage. They must be eliminated completely, for there is no benefit in partial reduction. That is a very strong statement, but if a cure has to be wrought we must eliminate everything that is definitely building up the blood-pressure. Other liquids harmful to this condition are tea,

coffee, milk, aerated waters and the very acid fruit juices. Even water itself, if taken too liberally, can bring about a certain increase in the blood-pressure. And so in the study of blood-pressure it appears that only the minimum of liquid is advisable, except when the urine becomes very concentrated, when a little more may be given.

The dry diet is naturally difficult at first, but if the temptation to drink is fought against, the desire will gradually diminish, especially when the diet becomes balanced. The abnormal thirst experienced by most people is very often due to the fact that their diet has been unbalanced and is creating certain digestive disturbances that are accompanied by thirst. A balanced diet prevents this and supplies a plentiful volume of distilled water in the vegetables and fruits.

BUILDING A DIET

Working from this basis we can now build an efficient health-giving and blood-pressure-reducing diet. First of all, on rising, if desired, an apple, orange, or pear may be taken. For breakfast fruit is best, either fresh acid or soaked and simmered dried fruit or occasionally tinned fruit, of which pineapple is the best variety. When the pressure is extremely high, the fruit should be limited to the milder sub-acid fruits such as apples, pears and grapes. Any kind of fruit, however, can be taken in most cases, such as apples, oranges, pears, grapes, grapefruit, lemons, plums, strawberries, raspberries, all tinned fruits, soaked and simmered prunes, apricots, figs and raisins. Dates are also good and may be taken at this breakfast meal. With the breakfast of fruit the varying fruit juices go well, and apple, orange, tomato, pineapple and grapefruit may be taken at this morning meal.

No other food or liquid should be taken at breakfast, because this often causes some form of digestive upset which would not arise if the fruit were taken by itself. It cannot be denied that the fruit and fruit juice breakfast is not a satisfying one at the beginning of the treatment, but usually it will be found that within a very short time this breakfast, a cleansing one that gradually rejuvenates the body, will be more appreciated than the one normally taken. It is only a matter of habit, and the person who persists with the fruit breakfast for a month will seldom, if ever, go back to the ordinary one.

The rest of the diet in high blood-pressure should consist in theory of two meals each with a basic salad composed of any fresh vegetables and fruits and with a small amount of protein at one meal and a small amount of starch at another. The fruit breakfast and the two salad meals, with protein and starch in very small quantities, form the ideal diet for all who suffer from increased arterial pressure.

So the lunch meal, if possible, should consist of a large salad, using lettuce, watercress, mustard and cress, grated cabbage, spinach, celery, carrots, turnips, tomatoes and every other kind of suitable vegetable. Fruit, such as dates, raisins, grapes, grated apple or pear, may be added. With this salad a small quantity of protein, such as lightly cooked egg, grated cheese or grated nuts, may be taken to make it more sustaining. In practice, it is advisable to leave the meal at that, and the person who is still hungry should take only dates or dates and raisins to satisfy the hunger. Taking any other kind of food, especially food of a starchy nature, reduces the benefit of this meal.

The evening meal should again be based on a large mixed vegetable and fruit salad, varied as much as possible from the lunch salad and with only olive oil, or olive oil and lemon juice, as a dressing. For the remainder of the meal some form of starch may be taken, for example, two or three small baked potatoes or two or three small slices of wholewheat bread, preferably homebaked, or oatcakes, crispbread, or digestive biscuits. This evening meal, the salad and starch meal, is often largely over-eaten, and a certain limit on the amount of starch is required. Naturally this is very difficult to assess because it varies with each person, but usually the meal should leave the appetite slightly unsatisfied.

The late evening meal should, in this scheme of treatment consist of fruit only. It is also very beneficial if the person who is going through this home treatment can take one day per week on fresh acid fruit and fruit juices only. One day on this very cleansing form of diet will do a great deal to bring down the blood-pressure, and it can be recommended with every confidence.

Some stout people will find that this dietary brings about a rapid reduction in weight, and yet in others there will be no great difference, although, generally speaking, the body does become smaller. This means that, with the reduction of liquid, there is an indrawing of the various tissues of the body and the person feels fitter in every way.

6.
Reactions to Diet

NOW THAT THE general diet has been outlined I wish to give you some idea of how the patient described in Chapter Four reacted to it. First of all, he was advised to take a fresh acid fruit breakfast comprising apples, pears, oranges and apple juice. There was no limit to the quantity of fruit, the important rule being that no other food or liquid was to be taken at this meal. As a result the patient felt hungry during the morning and was therefore inclined to take too much food at the lunch meal.

There was no effect, as far as could be ascertained, from the acid fruit breakfast for ten days. Then the patient began to feel that the oranges were too acid and that a certain amount of stomach acidity arose after they had been taken. They were replaced by grapes, which were digested normally. This breakfast was then found to be quite sustaining and beneficial, and had the definite effect of freshening the stomach. Before beginning this treatment, the patient had been aware that his digestive system was clogged and each morning his tongue had been dirty, but from the time the acid fruit breakfast was started until the first cleansing took place, the digestive tract was in a much healthier condition.

When the colder weather came, the patient was allowed to mix dried fruits such as prunes, figs, raisins and dried apples with the suitable acid fruits. A tablespoonful of crude black molasses was also given. This is not actually an ideal mixture, but it had the effect of giving something more sustaining. About three weeks after the beginning of the fruit breakfast, the patient was troubled by ulceration in the mouth. This was a sign that a definite cleansing was taking place and, although disagreeable, it could be regarded as something positive.

For a few days the fresh fruits were reduced and more of the dried fruit such as prunes, figs, raisins and apricots were given. These fruits, when they have been soaked and simmered, regain a great deal of their natural alkaline state, and although they may be lacking in vitamins, they are definitely useful for introducing mineral salts. At this time it was also found that crude black molasses, which had been given to aid the mineral content of the body, and which had been tolerated very well, gave rise to digestive discomfort and had to be stopped. It is regrettable that many of these substances, which are in themselves very well balanced foods, cannot be tolerated by modern digestions.

Up to this time the breakfast was the only meal changed, and there had been a slow drop until the systolic pressure was 200 and the diastolic 140, with a differential of 60. After three weeks the other meals were changed quite quickly, and the lunch, which had up till then been a practically normal meal, consisted of the following.

Soup, which had been taken freely, meat, and all forms of flesh protein and fish were stopped. Egg and cheese dishes and vegetarian savouries were substituted. Vegetables were given liberally, usually two or three per meal, sometimes raw and sometimes steamed, but potatoes were limited to two each meal. The dessert after this meal was composed of raisins, grapes, apples or pears, and all very acid fruits were avoided. The patient again found that this meal was not very satisfying but admitted that he arose from the table feeling much lighter than normally; and during the afternoon, even while he felt the need for more food, he was mentally and physically more alert, except for occasional bouts of tiredness.

EFFECTS OF BALANCED DIET

When a balanced diet is introduced to a person who has been living on a non-balanced diet over a period of years, it is quite likely that there will be frequent bouts of tiredness. Normally the person is receiving stimulation from small snippets of food, and when he or she adopts a regulated diet it is quite common to find that the lack of stimulating food soon becomes apparent. This does not mean that the new diet is wrong, because perseverance has proved that, as the power to assimilate the new food increased, the body does not require to be continually jogged along. The same applies to drinking and smoking. On a poor diet there is a much greater inclination for a person to smoke or drink to excess, because the food is lacking in minerals and vitamins, and the tendency then is always to take something to supplement what is lacking. Once the new diet has become a habit it will be found that the desire to smoke or drink is much reduced.

Following this lunch meal it was found that our patient felt the need of a stimulant during the afternoon, and he was given yogurt and also some sugar in the form of dates. These are two useful foodstuffs which cleanse the kidneys, invigorate the bowel and yet make available a certain amount of energy.

Cleansing the system does not always mean an increase in bowel activity; indeed, it may be the reverse, because in many cases the bowel slows down. During this time, however, much of the injurious matter within or connected to the bowel wall is detached and prepared for elimination. Looking over this case history I found that up to this stage of the treatment the patient was inclined to be constipated. There had been a slight looseness of the bowels on starting the fruit breakfast, but as the diet changes progressed the bowel appeared to become more and more sluggish.

This is quite an interesting point because, at the time of writing, a patient undergoing treatment for high blood-pressure on a similar diet has been so troubled with a great acitivity of the bowel that the fruits have had to be reduced. This goes to prove that each person must experiment to find the suitable changes in food that will supply all that the body needs for assimilation and ultimate energy and also give vitamins, minerals and eliminative materials. The latter are needed to maintain the flow through the body of food inward and impurities outward.

STARCHY EVENING MEAL

The patient under consideration then made the final change in his diet, namely the evening meal. Now this meal had normally been of the solid type, and when it was reduced to a starchy one there was not the same feeling of loss, because the starchy foods are naturally bulky. He was given starch in the form of potatoes which were baked or steamed, wholewheat bread or any wholewheat product such as fruit cake or biscuits. The crispbreads were also included, and all this starch was added to a large mixed and continually varied salad, which, of course, naturally changed with the vegetables and fruit in season. There was little restriction in the choice of salad, and he was given a fairly free rein, except that he was not allowed his favourite salad dressing. He complained that salad without the ordinary dressing and salt was most uninteresting, but he was advised to persevere and within a week or two he admitted that he did not notice the lack of these condiments.

No liquids were included with the evening meal, but when the patient felt hungry, later, he was allowed some juice such as apple, orange or tomato. This giving of liquid – water, buttermilk, fruit juices, strained vegetable soup – is actually departing from the basis of the treatment in which we are trying to reduce the volume of liquid within the body. It must be allowed, however, at least during the first few weeks of changing the diet, because the bloodstream becomes rather congested and slows up and there is abnormal thirst. As the various factors correct themselves, it will be found that much of this desire to drink something will disappear, and the patient will find that the amount of liquid required by the body can easily be reduced. When this is done we have reached the first main change in the constituents of the bloodstream.

These are very important points, and I am describing what happened in this case to help people following the home treatment of high blood-pressure. It is, of course, impossible to foretell how each patient will react, but once the basic principles of Natural Healing are understood, each person can improvise correctly to suit his particular traits.

POWER REGAINED

Within a few weeks of beginning the full diet the patient, who had been very depressed mentally, felt in much better spirits, and appreciated that at last he had set foot on a definite path to health. There was a general uplifting, and this was noticeable in his posture and walk. He had the aura of a person who was becoming energized and whose bloodstream was reaching that stage in which power, whatever that power may be, was being regained. This feeling of returning health often heralds such a rise in the strength, vitality or energy, call it what you may, of the blood, that there comes a form of house-cleaning. In other words, the body rises in strength and flings off some of its accumulations.

This was stressed to the patient at the time, because forewarned is forearmed; and within a few days he suffered not exactly from a physical complaint, but from great depression. There appeared to be a cloud hanging over him, and actually it is possible for anyone who is dealing all the time with patients, in health and ill-health, to 'feel' such an aura of blackness. This was dealt with mainly by encouraging suggestion, and within another week it had lifted. His blood-pressure was then taken, and the systolic pressure was found to be 182 and the diastolic 128, with a differential of 54 — a general all-round drop.

This patient expected, however, that there would have been a greater decrease in the pressure, because he felt so much better. This is one reason why many practitioners do not actually give details of the blood-pressure. It is not wise for the patient to be told the pressure is up, then down, then up and so on, and to be kept wondering all the time what the final outcome will be. His blood-pressure should always be related to his general health. If the pressure is failing and his health increasing, the actual fall of the pressure need not be of great significance. It is the general finding that the pressure is falling and the health of the body increasing that we are concerned about, and we must not put too much stress on figures. We must look on the body as a whole. When there is a tendency to a more positive physical, mental and emotional state, then a fall in pressure, be it ever so slight, is definitely a beneficial sign, and much more so than a very rapid fall in pressure without any appreciable improvement in general health.

If therefore, the patient is made aware of the actual pressures — and this certainly gives the intelligent patient a great deal of interest — these pressures should be drawn in the form of a graph which should show a decline in the systolic pressure and a slower decline in the diastolic pressure. These naturally vary with each patient and the condition of the arteries and veins, but roughly these are the directions which the lines of the graph should follow.

DIGESTIVE UPSET
This chapter has described the main changes that take place when the actual diet has been started, and it can be confidently expected that similar changes will occur in

most cases of people undergoing the home treatment of high blood-pressure. If any difficulty arises it is advisable to check if each individual article of the diet is suitable. If, for instance, some digestive upset follows the use of a certain food, that food should naturally be stopped, even though it may have beneficial qualities. It may be tried again later, and it often happens that a person who, for instance, cannot take an egg without suffering from biliousness immediately afterwards, can take eggs without discomfort when the diet is balanced.

Digestive upset, however, must be expected in some form or another with a total change of diet, because the foods that are advised are essentially foods that have not been taken before in any great quantity or particularly in suitable combination. In other words, if the patient had been living on this diet before he would not now be suffering from high blood-pressure. Nature Cure is not strictly limited to actual healing; it is also a method of living. We believe that it is the correct method because the food is given in balanced quantities, but the beginner in Nature Cure will, in most cases, suffer from some degree of digestive disturbance. It is better, therefore, for one who is not under the guidance of a practitioner, to stop the food or liquid that seems to be causing the trouble. Stop it for a week or two and then try it again, and it will often be found that on the second occasion it is better tolerated.

There is a gradual change in the chemistry of the blood during this treatment. It is usually reckoned that the change reaches its apex between the seventh and ninth week, and with it comes the power to utilize more and more of the foods that are difficult to digest. The digestion of difficult foods makes for a strong digestive system, in the same way that an arm is made strong by lifting heavy weights or by doing a great number of physical movements. So the digestive tract is forced to become active and healthy, and the body receives (which in most cases it has never received before) mineral salts that are of the utmost value to the chemistry of the bloodstream. Whenever Nature Cure is started, a great number of changes are set going in the system, and every one of these changes has some positive ending.

This is a most important point, and I do not wish anyone suffering from high blood-pressure and following the system outlined here to become dismayed when a disagreeable symptom arises. It is very difficult to understand the reactions that take place in the body; indeed, practitioners with years of experience are sometimes baffled by the various signs and symptoms that occur. During treatment all upsets of this nature must be treated by fasting on water only and resting as much as possible, and within hours or, at the most, a day or two, there will be a general clearing of the condition. Everyone suffers from poor circulation here or poor circulation there, and an accident, a birth injury or wrong posture can bring about conditions which in cleansing give rise to most peculiar symptoms.

THE GOLDEN RULE

So this is the golden rule. If you are puzzled and cannot get in touch with a naturopath, then you should fast and rest. In every case, of course, it is preferable if a practitioner can be contacted, because personal supervision should attempt to treat the body along the lines that have been outlined. If suppressive measures are used, much more harm than good will result. Nature Cure is an eliminative treatment, and the body will attempt to heal by elimination, by a tissue cleansing, by what is called the 'Nature Cure crisis'. It may be said in passing that this is a very ill-chosen title. It is not a crisis in any sense of the word; it is a cleansing that should be welcomed, and the patient who understands what is happening will approach it in such a way that the positivity that arises in the bloodstream from the cleansing will reduce any disagreeable symptoms to a minimum.

All cleansings of this nature, whether they come as fevers, catarrhal discharges, skin outbreaks or any form of inflammation, should be accepted willingly as a necessary part in the elimination of something within the body that is destructive. Before each cleansing that is of a positive nature there comes a feeling that the body is gaining in strength. That means a Nature Cure cleansing. If there is any upset of a destructive nature, the person does not feel well beforehand. Then there is a feeling of tiredness and loss of energy, and the power. These actual findings may occur immediately before any house-cleansing, but before that again there has been a feeling of aliveness, a feeling of returning health, and other people will have noticed this and will have remarked to the person that he is gaining in health. Then comes the tissue cleansing.

7.
Skin Elimination

BEFORE EXCESSIVE BLOOD-PRESSURE has reached the very serious stage, the general picture of the arterial system is of congestion; and in this chapter certain methods will be outlined which are designed to remove this tendency. In nearly every case the person suffering from extreme pressure is full of vitality, and doubtless this is an expression of congestion of the system; and by becoming mentally and physically active the sufferer obtains relief.

There are, of course, other methods of relieving the tension within the arterial system, and the foregoing diet will undoubtedly have aided greatly in this direction. It can be confidently stated that no sufferer from high blood-pressure can have followed this treatment so far without a reduction in the systolic pressure. The reduction, of course, will vary with each person and with many other factors such as occupation, nervous tension and the inclination to worry that goes with certain temperaments. All these things come into consideration, but if the treatment has been followed so far there will be a drop in the pressure, varying from ten to thirty points, in this short course.

It is not altogether wise, of course, to bring about a rapid drop in blood-pressure because the system has to make various changes and, generally speaking, a slow drop in all the pressures is desirable. Although the treatment so far will have brought about this reduction, it is a limited treatment and the rate of healing can be increased by stimulating the activity of the eliminating organs. Naturally the diet will have activated the bowel and kidneys; and the next important eliminating organ that we must study is the skin, which has been practically untouched by the methods already outlined.

The skin has the power to rid the body of considerable, although naturally varying, amount of impurity, and if we can devise methods whereby the skin becomes more active and effective in its action, the congestion within the body will be relieved. Naturally, when the skin is mentioned, most people think that the great elimination can be attained from very hot applications, and the Turkish bath comes to mind. This is a very strenuous method of forcing the skin to work, and it is certainly not advised for people who have very high blood-pressure. It is much safer to build up a system of skin hygiene that will increase the activity of this tissue over a period of time.

Nearly every skin is choked by the presence of millions of dead cells. This means that the skin has become very much thickened and engorged and that the normal interflow of the various substances through it has been reduced. One way to bring about activity in such a skin is to rub it vigorously with a dry, rough towel. This removes millions of useless cells, and this action can be made more effective if a cold wet towel is used. In this way the circulation in the skin is invigorated both by the friction and by the reaction to cold which brings about an extra blood-supply to the skin.

MASSAGE

This form of stimulation of the skin can be further increased if massage is employed. This massage should be performed by a skilled operator who knows exactly the movements that bring about drainage of the skin and of the lymphatic vessels below this tissue. Such treatment should be obtained regularly, and it should really aim at thinning the skin tissues rather than retoning the muscles. If it is performed by a naturopath, he will frequently use artificial sun-ray treatment at the same time; that is, the skin will be massaged beneath the rays from the sun-lamp.

This is a very stimulating treatment but it must be performed under professional guidance, because too much sun-ray, in the case of a person suffering from high blood-pressure, can be quite dangerous.

The person suffering from hypertension should seldom, if ever, sunbathe because it is easy to over-expose, and this means that the skin, for the time being, is out of action. Such an occurrence can, by reducing the function of the skin (a function that is never really noticed), increase the blood-pressure, and this may have quite serious consequences. If sun-bathing is indulged in at all it should be of extremely short duration, one or two minutes, and no attempt should be made to create a sun-tan.

If massage cannot be obtained it is possible to stimulate the skin by other methods, and here the salt glow treatment is most useful. In this, a handful of salt should be placed in a basin of water and dissolved slightly until it forms a 'snow'. This is rubbed fairly briskly all over the body, taking care that the abrasive action of the salt does not irritate a sensitive skin. After the salt has been allowed to dry on the skin and become slightly sticky, it is washed off with warm water. This is followed by a quick cold sponge down, if the person feels strong enough, and a brisk friction rub. This salt glow is most useful in increasing the eliminative action of the skin, and it can normally be taken about twice weekly, provided, of course, that the sensitive skin is not irritated by the salt. These factors must be taken into account, for many patients feel that the salt glow, although invigorating, irritates the skin. The treatment becomes more efficacious if Epsom salt is used, because this has a greater osmotic action.

CLEANSING THE SKIN

For general cleansing of the skin there is nothing to equal the warm soapy sponge-down followed by a plain warm-water rinse, then cold water and a brisk friction rub with a towel. This rub-down, especially if performed morning and night, will by itself reduce pressure. This has been proved by our records. This water treatment removes from the skin many poisonous substances that are coming within the body and clogging the pores. It is the best form of cleansing the skin, because the person who suffers from high blood-pressure should never take very hot baths. There is naturally a desire for such baths in people who have this trouble, because they are appreciated as a form of relaxation and in theory should be very helpful. It is possible, however, to weaken the skin action so much by hot baths that the skin becomes inactive, and in this way such baths bring about an increase in pressure.

The best plan is to stop all hot baths and limit the cleansing of the skin to the warm soapy sponge-down and the salt glow. Cold water bathing is not advised. Many people believe that a complete cold bath each morning will bring the body back to health. In high blood-pressure the shock of such a bath may result in arterial breakage, and it should be avoided until the pressure becomes normal. A cold sponge-down is of benefit in cases where the pressure is not abnormally high, but it is better if it has been preceded by the warm soapy sponge-down, which has a cleansing action and which also opens the pores and allows more expression. The cold water tends always to close the pores, although it has the benefit of increasing the circulation in the actual skin area. The person suffering from high blood-pressure should not subject himself to any severe water treatment, unless it is conducted under strict supervision.

Naturally in treating the efficiency of the skin, clothing comes very much into the picture, and the person who is inclined to wear very heavy clothing is doing a great deal of harm to the skin, because it is never allowed to 'breathe'. Ideally, underclothes should be of silk, linen or one of the porous types now obtainable. These allow the skin to disgorge its impurities and gaseous products. Where woollen underwear is used there is a tendency for the skin to be in a continual state of mild perspiration, and this is not always beneficial to the health. It is not possible, however, for people especially when elderly, to change these habits completely, and the usual method advised is to reduce the weight of underclothes gradually, especially during the spring. Very lightweight underclothes should be used during the summer, and slightly heavier ones during the next winter. I know this is not always suitable, but the general tendency should be towards lightness and to keeping the skin in a dry condition. Thinness and dryness are the two factors that must be associated with a healthy skin.

During Nature Cure treatment of high blood-pressure it is quite possible that the skin will discharge vigorously; that is, some kind of skin outbreak may occur. These outbreaks are helpful because they show that underneath there has been some form of impurity, and because of the renewed activity in the skin this impurity is being reduced. This cleansing of the body through the skin should be encouraged and never suppressed by the use of ointments, poultices or internal medication. It is very unlikely that this activity will be prolonged, and it will usually disappear quickly on a balanced diet. Outbreaks of the skin can usually be controlled by reducing the amount of starch and sugar in the diet. A milk diet is also of benefit in some forms of skin outbreak, but, of course, in the condition of high blood-pressure it should be used only for a short period because it increased the amount of fluid in the body.

SCALP AND FEET

In connection with the skin I would like to draw the attention of the reader to two very important parts, namely the scalp and the feet. For sufferers from high blood-pressure drainage of the scalp is very important, and general attention here will relieve many cases. The hair and scalp should, whenever possible, be washed at least once weekly, using plain soap. All forms of medicated shampoos and soaps should be avoided. The hair should be thoroughly rinsed after washing, and then the water should be cooled down before the final rinse. There is no need to take a cold head douche at the end of the washing, because this may upset the blood balance, but certainly the water should be cooled down until it is slightly cold. If this is done each week it will often result in a gradual increase in the dandruff. This is a sign that the scalp is really throwing out and acting in a normal way. If the treatment is continued the amount of dandruff will gradually be reduced, but while it is coming away it should be regarded as a helpful sign and never suppressed by any form of medication.

The feet are also excellent eliminators, and most of us discharge a considerable amount of impurity through the skin pores of these parts. The feet should therefore be washed at least once daily in warm, soapy water, followed by a rinsing in warm water and then a quick cold douche. If the feet perspire rather readily they should be treated in this fashion twice daily. In this way much of the impurity of the body is sent to the outside, and the person definitely feels relieved in every way. Stockings or socks should be changed frequently, and once daily is a very good plan in people who suffer from excessive perspiration in these extremities. On the other hand it is never wise to apply any form of suppressive medication for foot perspiration. Even the use of talcum powder can definitely be suppressive and harmful to the body as a whole, and its use should be stopped because the feet are part of the excretory system and as such should always be encouraged to eliminate.

Continuing our study of the person who started with a systolic pressure of 252 and a diastolic of 170, and whose pressure had fallen so many points by the time the diet had been thoroughly instituted, the following water treatments were advised for the skin. First of all, the warm, soapy sponge-down followed by a warm sponge and then a coldish sponge, was started each morning, and this was continued for a week, at the end of which a considerable improvement had taken place in the skin condition. It must be remembered that this patient was also having some treatment at the same time, including special massage and sun-ray; that contributed towards his improvement.

During the second week the patient was advised to have an Epsom salts bath. This bath had rather a peculiar effect, because it left the patient very stiff and sore next morning. This stiffness is usually a sign that the osmotic action of the Epsom salts is bringing impurities nearer the skin into some certain muscular groups. From the third week the patient was given a warm, soapy sponge-down in the morning, and three days of that week he was advised to have a salt glow at some other time during the day. He was also given one Epsom salt bath weekly. This was a fairly strenuous treatment for a person in poor physical condition, and at the end of a month he felt rather upset.

This was a natural reaction, and when it was explained to him he more or less cheered up and set about treatment with more gusto. As a result it was found that by the end of the eighth week, on the same diet as has been explained in the foregoing chapter, his systolic blood-pressure was 158 and his diastolic pressure 106, the differential being 52.

This was really a remarkable drop from the first recording, and it was also shown in the general demeanour of the patient. Everything about him was showing signs of health. He was more alert and more optimistic, and his whole outlook towards his trouble had changed. He was inclined if anything to become too enthusiastic about his cure. That is one of the dangers of Nature Cure. The person who is undergoing treatment, and who has the self-discipline to carry it out as far as possible, often becomes really too enthusiastic. Practitioners usually warn such patients that an eliminative house-cleansing often follows this sign of returning to health.

8.
Deep Breathing and Other Exercises

SEVERAL YEARS AGO a book was published explaining a treatment for high blood-pressure based solely on deep-breathing exercises. At that time I was particularly interested in this trouble, and outlined this course to several patients. Some of them were on a fairly strict diet, but others were only given the various breathing exercises, and a careful check was kept of the two different methods of treatment. The results were quite surprising. The patients who were on a diet similar to the one outlined in this book made rapid general progress and they all recorded a considerable reduction in their blood-pressure. On the other hand, the patients who practised deep-breathing exercises, without any other change in their method of living, at first showed considerable progress in reducing their pressures. This progress was convincing for about six weeks, but after this it was found that the pressures remained constant.

Following this, two other groups of patients were tried on slightly different lines. All of them were placed on a diet, but the second group also practised the deep-breathing exercises. The pressures of the first group fell rather slowly, but those of the group on the diet, aided by deep-breathing exercises, showed a considerable drop, and this was maintained until the pressure became approximately normal. This proves that there is a considerable advantage in practising deep-breathing exercises, especially if the rest of the treatment outlined in this book is followed.

One great difficulty in the practice of deep breathing is that a system of this kind tends to become monotonous, and usually it is found that the number of times the exercises are performed is gradually reduced until they are of no benefit. One way of getting round this difficulty is to do the exercises to music, and suitable records can be obtained. Another way is to practice deep breathing during a walk, and the added benefit of increased blood circulation is then obtained.

Exhalation — that is, breathing out or emptying the lungs — is the most important part of the deep-breathing movement. This ensures that many gaseous impurities are removed, and it also means that the emptying of the air is much increased. In walking and deep breathing, exhalation can be maintained for five or six steps and inhalation for four steps. The exhalation in this case requires some physical effort, but this is counter-balanced by the fact that the air is allowed to flow into the lungs and not forced in.

Practising deep breathing during walking is not an exercise that can be carried out for a long time. Within a few minutes it will be found that the oxygen content becomes very much increased, and then a deep breath can only be taken with difficulty and normal breathing must be resumed. This is a most important point, because many people become distressed when they find that they cannot breathe more deeply, but this is the natural reaction of the mechanism of the brain to reduce the amount of oxygen in the blood. There are, in addition to this, several exercises that can be performed at home. These are very simple, but they will bring about a great benefit and help very much in relieving the tension that is always present in cases of excessively high blood-pressure.

EXERCISE ONE
Lie on the back with knees bent and shoulders and head

supported by a cushion. Relax all muscles, then breathe slowly but deeply in through the nose, allowing the air to flow to the lower parts of the lungs. In doing so, the abdomen is pushed downwards, and it should give the appearance also of rising above the lower level of the chest. It is essential that the air is allowed to flow to the bottom of the lungs. When the lower lung is fully filled with air, hold this position for a few seconds and then slowly contract the abdomen and lower ribs, exhaling deeply at the same time. This exercise should be continued until slightly fatigued.

EXERCISE TWO

Stand erect. Take a deep breath through the nose and bend slowly to the right, pushing the right hand down the outside of the leg and raising the left arm above the head so that it can be used to lever the body to the right. As the movement is continued, breath should be slowly drawn inwards. Now bend to the left, and allow the left hand to come down the left leg, and right arm to come over the head, to lever the body over to the left. During this movement, breathe out. Continue in this fashion, breathing in as you bend to the right and out as you bend to the left, until there is a slight feeling of weariness. Then the sequence of breathing should be changed: Breathe in as you bend to the left and out when bending to the right. This exercise is designed primarily to bring about increased circulation in each lung, because with the bending of the body the movement of the lung is definitely retarded. It is an excellent exercise to increase the drainage of the lungs and to stimulate their eliminative action. It should be practised morning and night until slightly fatigued.

EXERCISE THREE

Stand erect with hands on the spine at the level of the

waist, fingers pointing towards the front of the body and thumbs actually on the spinal bones. Close mouth firmly, and then take in air in small amounts as if sniffing flowers. Continue to pack the lungs until no more can be taken. As you breathe in, bend the body gradually backward. When the chest is full, expel air slowly through the mouth, and at the same time bring the body to the bending-forward position. This exercise requires considerable practice, because it will be found that at first only a small amount of air can be be taken into the lungs; but within a week or two of daily practice it will be found that the capacity of the lungs is greatly increased. There is no limit to the number of times that this exercise should be done, but the rule is that the body should feel slightly fatigued before the exercise is stopped.

Naturally there are many exercises for increasing the capacity of the lungs, but these three and the breathing practised during walking will suffice to increase the lung capacity, drain the lung tissues and help very much in the removal of catarrhal deposits which are often found in cases of high blood-pressure. Remember that in this condition a certain amount of chokage or congestion throughout the whole body is common, and if the lungs can be stimulated into a healthier state much is being done to increase the rate of combustion and remove impurities from the body. In the case of the person with high blood-pressure whose transit towards health has been discussed, these four breathing exercises were started about the tenth week of treatment and resulted in a slight drop in blood-pressure within a few days. Within fourteen days his blood-pressure read as follows: Systolic, 148; diastolic, 100; differential, 48.

By this time it had become obvious to the patient that if he obeyed all the rules and performed the exercises explained in this chapter, his blood-pressure would come back to normal. This, of course, gave an added incentive, and his diet was kept on a very simple basis and he performed his exercises with integrity.

One point that worries many patients is deciding how long these exercises should be performed. This depends greatly on the condition of the patient and on the time at his or her disposal. Once when examining a patient who had been suffering from very high blood-pressure I asked him about the time he spent on exercising. He had found that he could practice the deep-breathing and walking part of the régime going to the office, and therefore he deliberately arranged to walk a certain distance each morning doing the exercise at this time. In all, this took about fifteen minutes. During the evening he allowed himself an hour's rest after the last meal, and then he practised the other breathing exercises for about ten minutes. He admitted that on certain nights he did not feel like exercising, but he persevered and very often found himself much refreshed after the movements had been performed. About half an hour per day is a general rule for the time to be spent exercising. Of course, a person with more time to be spent on his hands could increase the exercise with quite considerable benefit. This patient also remarked that in addition to the great benefit of a very much reduced blood-pressure, there was an appreciable improvement in his circulation, especially in his hands, which had always been cold in the winter. The Nature Cure diet, with its low starch content, often results in a patient feeling colder during the first winter of treatment. This is generally remedied in the second winter, but deep-breathing exercises can be of great benefit in all cases of poor circulation.

STRENUOUS MOVEMENT HARMFUL

It is usual to find that the sufferer from high blood-pressure has been warned not to indulge in excessive physical effort, and bending and lifting heavy weights are very definitely ruled out by most physicians. On reading this chapter about breathing exercises readers therefore may be tempted to ignore such advice and to start all manner of movements. This is definitely not advised. All strenuous movements, especially those including bending, will certainly do more harm than good. The blood-pressure must be almost normal before exercises of this type are attempted. Walking with deep breathing and the other breathing exercises described are in a totally different category. They are 'safe' exercises, and provided the person does not overtire physically they will always be beneficial.

When the blood-pressure is very high a certain strain is placed on the heart, and then walking up the slightest incline brings about a feeling of tightness in the chest. This is a definite warning and it must be heeded. It will usually be found that if the person affected rests and then resumes slow walking, the tightness will gradually disappear. This should always be the technique employed if such an attack occurs. The diet and other methods described in this book will bring about an invigoration of the heart and blood-vessels, and it can be expected that this tightness about the chest will gradually disappear. It must be remembered that the heart is only a specialized muscle and, like every other muscle in the body, requires to be kept in tone. The sufferer from high blood-pressure who has been taking some care and doing little exercise must also retone his heart muscles when he again begins to exercise. Slow walking with deep breathing over level ground is an excellent beginning. After a short time the heart will begin to pump the blood more forcibly, and then slight inclines may be attempted gradually until walks over quite steep inclines can be negotiated without difficulty. This gradual increase in the power of the heart muscle is very desirable, and it must be studied by all who find that tightness in the chest accompanies high blood-pressure.

In passing, it may be stated that a feeling of gripping in the chest is not always a sign that he heart is affected, and often this symptom comes from a flatulent condition in the stomach. The dry diet described in another chapter ensures mastication of food and often removes this symptom. Flatulence, however, also follows the eating of a large amount of vegetables, and this presents another slight difficulty in certain cases. Generally speaking, uncooked vegetables are better than cooked for this symptom, and if they are thoroughly masticated very little flatulence will become evident. The digestion of vegetables is not easy, and when a person has been living on a comparatively low vegetable diet the stomach and bowel are unused to dealing with such food. A few weeks on the diet outlined will remove this tendency, and nearly every vegetable will be digested without upset. When, however, flatulence is severe, it will be found that baked potatoes and well toasted wholewheat bread taken with the vegetables will bring some relief.

Normally when a person suffers from flatulence there is a tendency to take some form of alkaline powder such as sodium bicarbonate, but in Natural Healing no form of medication is advised. We think that everything introduced to the body via the mouth should be a food or liquid that will be of benefit to the body at some stage. Alkalies of the nature mentioned are not foods, and although they may result in a reduction of the flatulence within the bowel their after-effects can be harmful.

Once the blood-pressure has become near normal, mild exercises of a general nature can be taken, but naturally all movements that can upset the heart-beat must be regulated. Exercises that relax, rather than contract, are the most desirable. In my opinion, in addition to breathing exercises, every effort should be made to relieve any neck tension, and this can be achieved by the following two exercises which may be added to the daily routine.

EXERCISE ONE
Stand erect. Imagine that a pointer is being held just in

front of the nose and practice rolling the nose round the tip of this pointer, describing a very small circle with the head. This should be done moving the nose to the right for a few minutes and then to the left. This movement exercises the smaller group of neck muscles.

EXERCISE TWO

Stand erect, then roll the head (relaxing the muscles as much as possible) to the right completing the full circle. When this exercise is performed correctly, it should be felt that the neck is loose on he shoulders. After completing a few turns roll the head to the left. These two exercises can be practised at any time and are of great benefit in removing the neck tension that arises from physical and emotional strain.

These six exercises are the essentials for all cases of blood-pressure and they should be practised faithfully each day.

9.
The Cold Compress

IN NATURAL HEALING the reaction of the cold compress is often used to stimulate the action of the kidneys. This is a very safe method, and provided the desired reaction is obtained it will help the elimination of impurities and, by doing so, reduce the blood-pressure. Many sufferers from this trouble are afraid that the initial reaction to cold may be harmful, but this is always local, and compresses can be applied to all but the very serious cases. However, it is better to give some ruling in this matter, and it could be said that compressing should not be used, without professional guidance, when the systolic pressure is above two hundred.

The actual compress itself consists of a piece of linen which should be of a length to encircle the body once and overlap one inch for fastening. The breadth of this compress varies, but the general rule is that it should be in the region of eight inches, although it can be made much broader to reach from the ribs to the waist. This compress is soaked in cold water, wrung out and then applied to the waist area in such a way that its upper part covers the lower three ribs. Once applied, it can be fastened with safety pins and then covered completely with two or even three layers of woollen or flannel material to retain the reaction in the compress.

The desired reaction is a feeling of warmth in the skin beneath the compress, and it usually takes place about fifteen to twenty minutes after the compress has been applied. When this reaction is obtained the result will always be beneficial. If the compress remains cold it should be removed and the skin of the part sponged with warm water and dried by brisk towelling. The reaction to the cold compress varies considerably with each person, and even when a compress has been reacting it is common to find that suddenly the reaction is lost. If this happens, compressing should be stopped for several nights and then tried again. Compresses are usually applied just before retiring, and it is likely that they will be completely dry in the morning. The linen should be boiled after each application because the impurities are drawn through the skin during the reaction.

Although the skin of the part covered by the compress is invigorated, the desired reaction takes place deep in the tissues. This brings an immediate increase in the strength of the blood-flow in all the parts covered, and the congestion is reduced.

Many patients find the idea of applying a compress rather unpleasant but it is such a soothing and sleep-producing treatment that they soon become accustomed to it and finally are disinclined to stop it. Compressing is best carried out for about two months at a time and can be applied five nights weekly. It should then be stopped for at least one month, after which the treatment can be recommenced. This is the ideal treatment for people who find that the rate of fall of the blood-pressure has slowed down and seems to require a new impetus.

Sufferers must not become despondent if their pressure remains high. As stated before, Natural Healing is an all-round treatment and every tissue of the body is affected by its action. In other words, the health of the arterial system is always increased, and this alone makes it more capable of withstanding stresses and strains and the danger of breakage becomes more and more remote.

How a person looks and feels is a much better guide to the condition of the tissues than most of us really understand, and readers who have followed the tenets outlined in this book will undoubtedly have benefited in many ways. The cleansing of the bloodstream and the reduction of the accompanying nervous tension means that the whole outlook to health assumes a new aspect.

CONTROL OF THOUGHTS

Health is a matter of mind and body. Control of thoughts at a positive level is aided very much by the type of food introduced into the body. Yet the cultivating of uplifting and relaxing thoughts come within the control of everyone and, needless to say, this plays a great part in the treatment of high blood-pressure. Relaxation through thought-control should be studied by every sufferer, but it is usual to find that the active, physical type who usually suffer from high blood-pressure do not appreciate this and confine their relaxation to some change of energy. This is very wrong, and these sufferers are earnestly advised to cultivate more moderate mental activities to bring about relaxation.

Although I have attempted in this book to give some idea of the control of high blood-pressure through diet and exercises, it must not be assumed that this is all that is meant by the term Nature Cure. This is very far removed from the actual fact, and to every reader I would advise that the books written about this subject should be studied at length. It is only by doing so that the real meaning of Nature Cure will be understood in all its facets.

To the sufferer from serious high blood-pressure I would first of all advise that this book be read again with the purpose of understanding each change in the treatment. Some thought should be given to the reasons for the various steps, because with this understanding comes the determination to follow the advice implicitly, and that is the only way to success.

Once the main trend of the treatment is understood the treatment should be commenced immediately, and assuredly within a few weeks the general lightening of spirit which comes with all positive measures will be appreciated.

Finally, in this treatment it is never wise to study daily improvements, and it is best to calculate the progress made at some two-monthly intervals. Looking back over each of these periods, a very marked improvement in the physical condition will be seen, and then the progression of the treatment can be approached with every confidence.